DASH DIET MEAL PREP FOR CHRONIC KIDNEY DISEASE

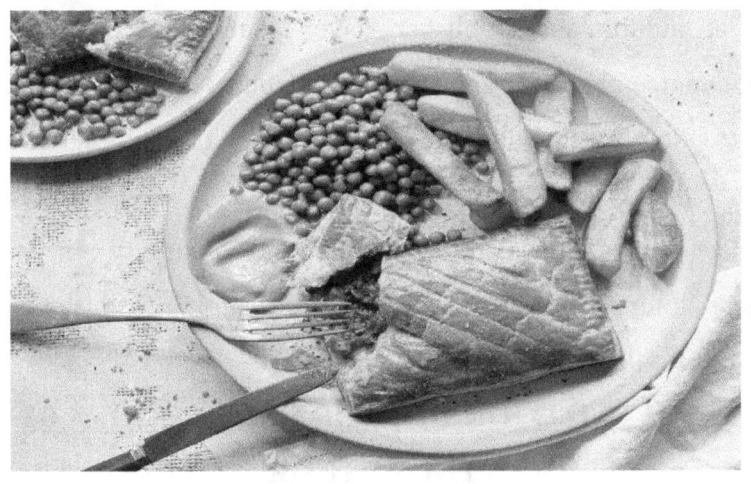

"60 Nutritious DASH Diet Recipes to Improve Renal Function and Health"

Harley Kemp

Copyright © 2024 by Harley Kemp
All rights reserved.

No part of this publication may be reproduced, stored in a retrieval system, or transmitted in any form or by any means, electronic, mechanical, photocopying, recording, or any other without the prior written permission of the copyright holder, except for brief quotations in critical reviews or articles.

The author and publisher have taken every effort to guarantee the accuracy and completeness of the material provided in this book. Nevertheless, they cannot guarantee that the information is free from mistakes, omissions, or inaccuracies, nor can they accept responsibility for any loss, injury, or damage caused by or resulting from the use of this book.

SCAN AND LOOK OUT FOR OTHER BOOKS BY THE AUTHOR

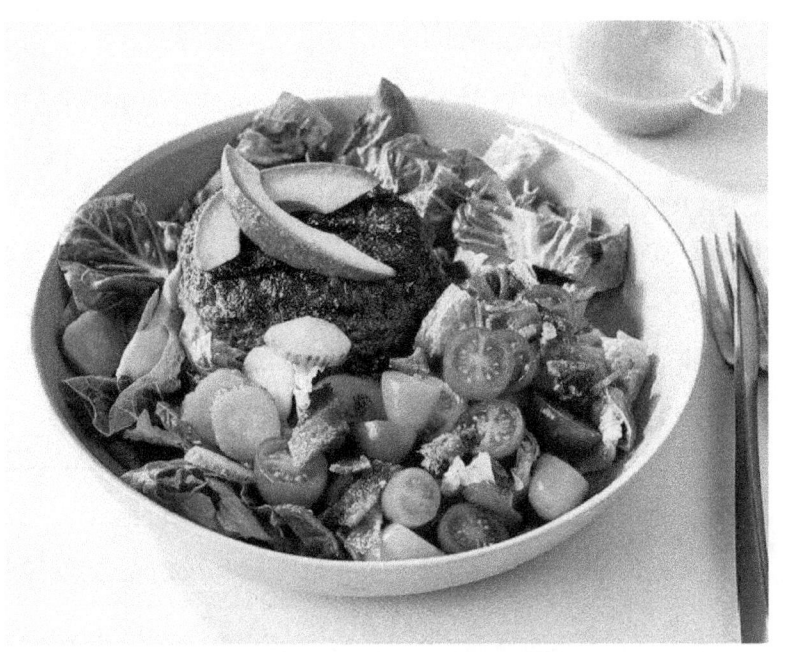

TABLE OF CONTENTS

INTRODUCTION 9

CHAPTER 1: UNDERSTANDING CHRONIC KIDNEY DISEASE 10

    Introduction to Chronic Kidney Disease (CKD): 10

    Causes and Risk Factors: 10

    Stages of CKD: 11

    Importance of Diet in Managing CKD: 12

CHAPTER 2: INTRODUCTION TO THE DASH DIET 14

    What is the DASH Diet? 14

History and Background: 14

Scientific Basis for DASH Diet: 15

Benefits of DASH Diet for CKD Patients: 16

CHAPTER 3: NUTRITIONAL GUIDELINES FOR CKD AND DASH DIET 18

Key Nutrients for CKD Patients: 18

Tailoring the DASH Diet for CKD: 20

CHAPTER 4: MEAL PLANNING AND PREPPING BASICS 22

Importance of Meal Planning for CKD Patients: 22

Tips for Successful Meal Planning and Prepping: 23

Tools and Resources for Meal Prep: 24

CHAPTER 5: DASH DIET BREAKFAST RECIPES FOR CKD 27

1. Veggie and Cheese Egg Muffins: 27

2. Berry Quinoa Breakfast Bowl: 28

3. Greek Yogurt and Fruit Parfait: 29

4. Spinach and Feta Breakfast Wrap: 30

5. Peanut Butter Banana Smoothie: 31

6. Whole Wheat Pancakes with Berries: 31

7. Avocado Toast with Poached Egg: 33

8. Overnight Chia Seed Pudding: 34

9. Turkey and Veggie Breakfast Burrito: 35

10. Almond Butter and Banana Toast: 36

CHAPTER 6: LUNCH RECIPES **37**

1. Grilled Chicken Salad: 37

2. Quinoa and Black Bean Salad: 38

3. Tuna Salad Lettuce Wraps: 39

4. Vegetable Stir-Fry with Brown Rice: 40

5. Turkey and Avocado Wrap: 41

6. Lentil Soup: 42

7. Grilled Veggie Wrap: 43

8. Chicken and Vegetable Stir-Fry: 44

9. Mediterranean Chickpea Salad: 45

10. Egg Salad Lettuce Wraps: 46

CHAPTER 7: DINNER RECIPES **48**

1. Baked Salmon with Roasted Vegetables: 48

2. Turkey Chili: 49

3. Lemon Herb Grilled Chicken: 50

4. Vegetable Stir-Fry with Tofu: 51

5. Shrimp and Vegetable Skewers: 53

6. Baked Cod with Herbed Quinoa: 54

7. Beef and Vegetable Stir-Fry: 55

8. Stuffed Bell Peppers: 56

9. Veggie and Tofu Stir-Fry: 57

10. Lemon Garlic Shrimp Pasta: 58

CHAPTER 7: SNACK AND APPETIZER IDEAS 60

1. Hummus and Veggie Sticks: 60

2. Greek Yogurt Dip with Whole Grain Crackers: 61

3. Caprese Skewers: 62

4. Cucumber and Cream Cheese Roll-Ups: 63

5. Apple Slices with Almond Butter: 64

6. Cottage Cheese with Pineapple: 64

7. Edamame Hummus with Whole Grain Pita Chips: ... 65

8. Avocado Salsa with Baked Tortilla Chips: 66

9. Roasted Chickpeas: 67

10. Stuffed Mini Bell Peppers: 68

CHAPTER 8: DESSERTS RECIPES 70

1. Fruit Salad with Honey-Lime Dressing: 70

2. Greek Yogurt Parfait with Berries and Granola: 71

3. Baked Apples with Cinnamon and Walnuts: 71

4. Frozen Yogurt Bark with Mixed Nuts and Berries: .. 73

5. Chocolate Avocado Mousse: 74

6. Banana Oatmeal Cookies: 75

7. Chia Seed Pudding with Fresh Fruit: 76

8. Strawberry Banana Smoothie: 77

9. Almond Flour Blueberry Muffins: 78

10. Coconut Mango Rice Pudding: 79

CHAPTER 9: SMOOTHIE RECIPES 81

1. Green Power Smoothie: 81

2. Berry Blast Smoothie: 82

3. Tropical Paradise Smoothie: 83

4. Peanut Butter Banana Smoothie: 83

5. Creamy Avocado Smoothie: 84

6. Mixed Berry and Spinach Smoothie: 85

7. Mango Peach Smoothie: 86

8. Blueberry Banana Smoothie: 87

9. Cherry Almond Smoothie: 88

10. Raspberry Coconut Smoothie: 89

CHAPTER 10: FREQUENTLY ASKED QUESTIONS 90

Common Concerns and Queries about CKD and the DASH Diet.. 90

1. Can the DASH Diet benefit individuals with CKD?. 90

2. Is the DASH Diet suitable for all stages of CKD? 90

How does the DASH Diet help manage blood pressure in CKD? 91

Are there specific foods to avoid on the DASH Diet for CKD? 91

How can I incorporate the DASH Diet into my lifestyle if I have CKD? 92

Can the DASH Diet help slow the progression of CKD? 93

What role does hydration play in CKD and the DASH Diet? 93

How can I manage protein intake on the DASH Diet for CKD? 94

14-Day Meal Plan 95

CONCLUSION 100

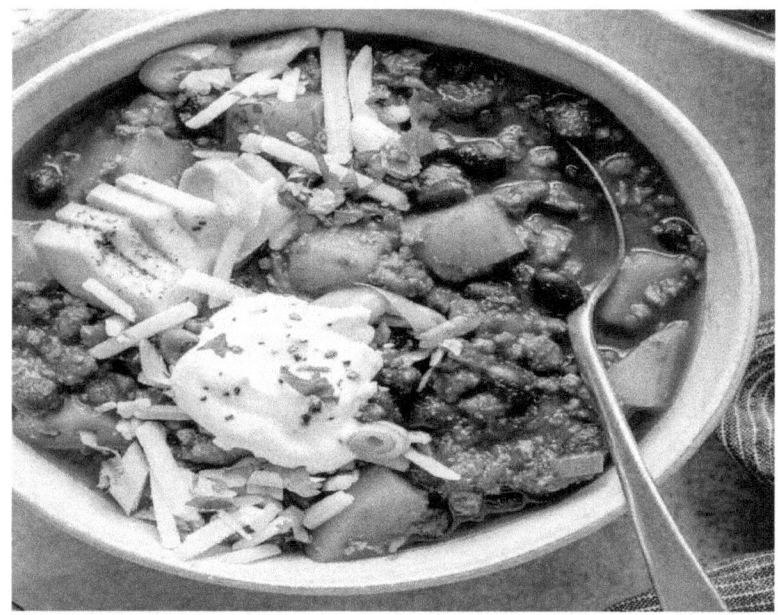

INTRODUCTION

Lena had been grappling with the challenges of Chronic Kidney Disease (CKD) for years. Fatigue, dietary restrictions, and the constant fear of worsening symptoms weighed heavily on her. Desperate for a solution, she stumbled upon the DASH Diet tailored for CKD. With cautious optimism, Lena embarked on her journey of meal prep and mindful eating. Slowly but steadily, she noticed changes. Her blood pressure stabilized, her energy levels soared, and her kidney function showed signs of improvement. What once felt like an insurmountable obstacle now seemed manageable. Lena found joy in discovering delicious recipes packed with kidney-friendly nutrients. Each meal became an opportunity to nourish her body and reclaim her health. With the DASH Diet as her guide, Lena's journey with CKD transformed from a struggle to a triumph, proving that with determination and the right dietary choices, a brighter, healthier future is within reach.

CHAPTER 1: UNDERSTANDING CHRONIC KIDNEY DISEASE

Introduction to Chronic Kidney Disease (CKD):

A degenerative illness known as chronic kidney disease (CKD) is characterized by a progressive loss of kidney function over time. In addition to manufacturing hormones that regulate numerous body functions, the kidneys are essential for filtering waste and extra fluid from the circulation and controlling blood pressure. When the kidneys are damaged or unable to function properly for an extended period, it leads to CKD.

Causes and Risk Factors:

Several factors can contribute to the development of CKD, including:

1. Diabetes: Uncontrolled diabetes is one of the leading causes of CKD. High blood sugar levels can damage the blood vessels in the kidneys, impairing their ability to filter waste effectively.

2. Hypertension (High Blood Pressure): Persistent high blood pressure can strain the blood vessels in the kidneys, causing damage over time.

3. Glomerulonephritis: Chronic kidney disease (CKD) can result from inflammation of the glomeruli, the kidney's filtering units

4. Polycystic Kidney Disease (PKD): A genetic condition known as polycystic kidney disease (PKD) is typified by the development of fluid-filled kidney cysts that can impede kidney function.

5. Other factors: Other conditions such as autoimmune diseases, kidney infections, urinary tract obstructions, and prolonged use of certain medications can also contribute to CKD.

Stages of CKD:

CKD is classified into five stages based on the estimated Glomerular Filtration Rate (eGFR), which measures how well the kidneys are filtering waste from the blood. The stages are as follows:

- **Stage 1:** Kidney damage with normal or high eGFR (≥ 90 mL/min/1.73 m^2)

- **Stage 2:** Mild decrease in eGFR (60-89 mL/min/1.73 m²)
- **Stage 3:** Moderate decrease in eGFR (30-59 mL/min/1.73 m²)
- **Stage 4:** Severe decrease in eGFR (15-29 mL/min/1.73 m²)
- **Stage 5:** Kidney failure (eGFR <15 mL/min/1.73 m² or on dialysis)

Importance of Diet in Managing CKD:

Diet plays a crucial role in managing CKD and slowing its progression. A well-balanced diet can help reduce the workload on the kidneys, control blood pressure and blood sugar levels, manage electrolyte imbalances, and prevent complications associated with CKD. Key dietary considerations for CKD patients include:

1. Sodium restriction: Limiting sodium intake helps control blood pressure and fluid retention, reducing the strain on the kidneys.

2. Potassium and phosphorus management: CKD patients may need to monitor their intake of potassium and phosphorus to prevent imbalances that can affect heart and bone health.

3. Protein moderation: Consuming an appropriate amount of high-quality protein can help preserve kidney function and prevent muscle wasting without overburdening the kidneys.

4. Fluid control: Monitoring fluid intake is essential for managing fluid retention and preventing complications such as edema and high blood pressure.

By adopting a kidney-friendly diet tailored to their individual needs and stage of CKD, patients can optimize their health outcomes, improve their quality of life, and better manage their condition in collaboration with their healthcare team.

CHAPTER 2: INTRODUCTION TO THE DASH DIET

What is the DASH Diet?

The Dietary Approaches to Stop Hypertension (DASH) diet is an eating plan designed to help lower blood pressure and reduce the risk of cardiovascular disease. Developed by the National Institutes of Health (NIH), the DASH diet emphasizes consuming a variety of nutrient-rich foods while limiting sodium, saturated fats, and cholesterol.

History and Background:

The DASH diet was developed through extensive research conducted by the NIH in the 1990s. The initial DASH study aimed to investigate the effects of dietary patterns on blood pressure, specifically focusing on the impact of diet on hypertension (high blood pressure). The findings from this study, along with subsequent research, demonstrated the efficacy of the DASH diet in reducing blood pressure and improving overall cardiovascular health.

Scientific Basis for DASH Diet:

The DASH diet is based on principles of balanced nutrition and emphasizes the following key components:

1. Fruits and vegetables: Rich in vitamins, minerals, and antioxidants, fruits and vegetables are central to the DASH diet. These foods provide essential nutrients while being low in calories and high in fiber, which supports heart health.

2. Whole grains: Whole grains such as brown rice, whole wheat bread, and oatmeal are sources of complex carbohydrates and fiber, which help regulate blood sugar levels and promote satiety.

3. Lean proteins: The DASH diet encourages lean protein sources such as poultry, fish, nuts, and legumes while limiting red meat and processed meats high in saturated fat and cholesterol.

4. Low-fat dairy: Dairy products are included in the DASH diet for their calcium and protein content, but emphasis is placed on choosing low-fat or fat-free options to reduce saturated fat intake.

5. Limited sodium: One of the distinctive features of the DASH diet is its emphasis on reducing sodium intake. High sodium consumption is associated with elevated blood pressure, so the DASH diet recommends limiting sodium to no more than 2,300 milligrams per day, with an ideal target of 1,500 milligrams per day for those with hypertension or at risk of developing it.

Benefits of DASH Diet for CKD Patients:

The DASH diet offers several potential benefits for individuals with Chronic Kidney Disease (CKD), including:

1. Blood pressure management: Hypertension is a common complication of CKD and can accelerate the progression of kidney damage. The DASH diet's focus on whole, nutrient-rich foods and limited sodium intake can help lower blood pressure and reduce the risk of further kidney damage.

2. Heart health: CKD patients are at increased risk of cardiovascular disease, and the DASH diet's emphasis on heart-healthy foods can help lower cholesterol levels, improve lipid profiles, and reduce the risk of heart disease.

3. Kidney function preservation: By promoting a balanced intake of nutrients and limiting potentially harmful substances like sodium and saturated fats, the DASH diet may help slow the progression of CKD and preserve kidney function over time.

4. Weight management: The DASH diet's emphasis on whole foods, fruits, vegetables, and lean proteins can support weight loss or weight maintenance goals, which is beneficial for CKD patients, as obesity is a risk factor for kidney disease progression.

Overall, the DASH diet offers CKD patients a well-rounded approach to nutrition that can complement medical treatment and lifestyle modifications aimed at managing their condition and improving their overall health outcomes.

CHAPTER 3: NUTRITIONAL GUIDELINES FOR CKD AND DASH DIET

Key Nutrients for CKD Patients:

1. Sodium:

- **Role:** Sodium plays a crucial role in maintaining fluid balance and regulating blood pressure. However, excessive sodium intake can lead to fluid retention and hypertension, both of which can exacerbate kidney damage in CKD patients.

- **Recommendation:** CKD patients should limit their sodium intake to help manage blood pressure and fluid retention. The recommended daily sodium intake varies but generally ranges from 1,500 to 2,300 milligrams per day, depending on individual health status and treatment goals.

2. Potassium:

- **Role:** Potassium is an essential mineral that plays a vital role in nerve function, muscle contraction, and maintaining fluid and electrolyte balance. However, impaired kidney function can lead to potassium

buildup in the blood, known as hyperkalemia, which can be dangerous.
- **Recommendation:** CKD patients may need to monitor their potassium intake to prevent hyperkalemia. Depending on their stage of CKD and individual health status, they may be advised to limit high-potassium foods such as bananas, oranges, potatoes, tomatoes, and dairy products.

3. **Phosphorus:**
   - **Role:** Phosphorus is involved in bone health, energy metabolism, and cell function. In CKD, impaired kidney function can lead to phosphorus retention in the blood, which can contribute to bone and cardiovascular complications.
   - **Recommendation:** CKD patients may need to limit their phosphorus intake, especially in later stages of the disease when kidney function is significantly impaired. This may involve reducing consumption of phosphorus-rich foods such as dairy products, nuts, seeds, whole grains, and processed foods with phosphate additives.

4. **Protein:**

- **Role:** Protein is essential for tissue repair, muscle growth, and overall health. However, excessive protein intake can put strain on the kidneys and may accelerate the progression of CKD.
- **Recommendation:** CKD patients should aim for a moderate protein intake tailored to their individual needs and stage of CKD. High-quality protein sources such as lean meats, poultry, fish, eggs, and plant-based proteins like beans and legumes are recommended. The amount of protein needed may vary but is generally lower than what is recommended for individuals with healthy kidneys.

Tailoring the DASH Diet for CKD:

To tailor the DASH diet to meet the needs of CKD patients, consider the following modifications:

1. Sodium restriction: Emphasize low-sodium alternatives and encourage the use of herbs, spices, and other flavor enhancers to reduce the need for added salt.

2. Potassium management: Monitor potassium intake and limit high-potassium foods as necessary, while still prioritizing a diet rich in fruits and vegetables low in potassium.

3. Phosphorus control: Be mindful of phosphorus intake and choose lower-phosphorus alternatives when possible, such as selecting dairy products with lower phosphorus content or opting for phosphorus-free additives.

4. Protein moderation: Adjust protein intake based on individual needs and stage of CKD, aiming for a moderate but adequate amount to support overall health while minimizing stress on the kidneys.

CHAPTER 4: MEAL PLANNING AND PREPPING BASICS

Importance of Meal Planning for CKD Patients:

Meal planning is essential for CKD patients for several reasons:

1. Nutritional management: Planning meals in advance allows CKD patients to ensure they are consuming a well-balanced diet that meets their nutritional needs while adhering to any dietary restrictions recommended by their healthcare team.

2. Sodium, potassium, and phosphorus control: CKD patients need to monitor their intake of sodium, potassium, and phosphorus to manage blood pressure, electrolyte balance, and mineral metabolism. Meal planning enables them to choose foods lower in these nutrients and control their intake more effectively.

3. Blood sugar management: For CKD patients with diabetes, meal planning plays a crucial role in managing blood sugar levels and preventing complications associated with fluctuating glucose levels.

4. Portion control: Controlling portion sizes is important for managing weight, blood pressure, and fluid retention in CKD patients. Meal planning helps individuals portion out their meals and snacks appropriately to avoid overeating.

Tips for Successful Meal Planning and Prepping:

1. Set realistic goals: Start by setting achievable goals for meal planning and prepping, considering factors such as time, budget, and dietary preferences.

2. Create a meal schedule: Establish a regular meal schedule with planned meals and snacks throughout the day to help maintain consistent blood sugar levels and prevent overeating.

3. Plan balanced meals: Aim to include a variety of foods from different food groups in each meal, focusing on lean proteins, whole grains, fruits, vegetables, and healthy fats.

4. Consider dietary restrictions: Take into account any dietary restrictions or recommendations provided by healthcare professionals, such as limiting sodium, potassium, or phosphorus intake, and tailor meal plans accordingly.

5. Make a shopping list: Before grocery shopping, create a list of ingredients needed for planned meals and snacks to ensure you have everything on hand when it's time to cook.

6. Batch cook and freeze: Cook larger batches of meals and portion them out into individual servings to freeze for later use. This makes it easier to have healthy, homemade meals on hand, especially on busy days.

7. Use convenient cooking methods: Choose cooking methods that require minimal time and effort, such as slow cooking, pressure cooking, or one-pan meals, to streamline meal preparation.

8. Incorporate leftovers: Plan meals that can easily be repurposed into leftovers for future meals, reducing food waste and saving time in the kitchen.

9. Stay organized: Keep track of meal plans, recipes, and grocery lists in a centralized location, such as a meal planning app or notebook, to stay organized and on track with your goals.

Tools and Resources for Meal Prep:

1. Meal planning apps: Utilize meal planning apps that offer features such as customizable meal plans, grocery lists, and recipe databases to simplify the meal planning process.

2. Recipe websites and cookbooks: Explore recipe websites and cookbooks that specialize in CKD-friendly recipes and meal ideas, providing inspiration and guidance for meal planning.

3. Food scales and measuring cups: Invest in kitchen tools such as food scales and measuring cups to accurately portion out ingredients and adhere to dietary recommendations.

4. Meal prep containers: Purchase reusable meal prep containers in various sizes to portion out meals and snacks ahead of time for easy storage and transport.

5. Nutrition labels: Learn how to read and interpret nutrition labels on packaged foods to make informed choices about sodium, potassium, phosphorus, and other nutrient content.

6. Support groups and online communities: Join CKD support groups and online communities where members share meal planning tips, recipes, and resources for managing their condition through nutrition.

By implementing these strategies and utilizing available tools and resources, CKD patients can effectively plan and prepare meals that support their health goals, enhance their well-being, and simplify the management of their condition.

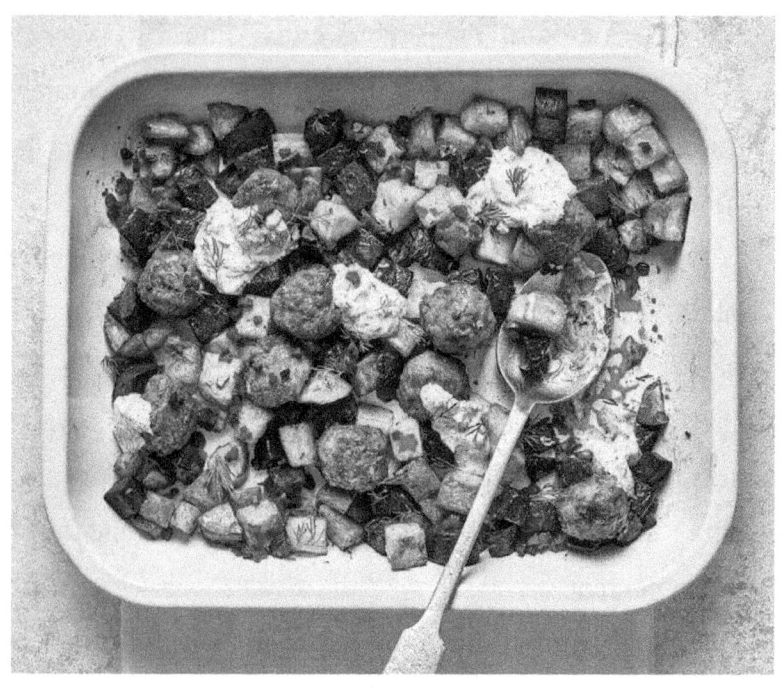

CHAPTER 5: DASH DIET BREAKFAST RECIPES FOR CKD

1. Veggie and Cheese Egg Muffins:

INGREDIENTS:

- 6 large eggs
- 1/4 cup diced bell peppers
- 1/4 cup diced onions
- 1/4 cup diced tomatoes
- 1/4 cup chopped spinach
- 1/4 cup shredded low-fat cheese
- Salt and pepper to taste

INSTRUCTIONS:

1. Preheat the oven to 350°F (175°C) and grease a muffin tin.

2. In a bowl, whisk together eggs, vegetables, cheese, salt, and pepper.

3. Pour the egg mixture evenly into the muffin tin.

4. Bake for 20-25 minutes or until the muffins are set and lightly golden.

PREP TIME: 10 MINUTES

Nutritional Values (per serving):

- Calories: 100
- Protein: 8g
- Carbohydrates: 2g
- Fat: 6g

2. Berry Quinoa Breakfast Bowl:

INGREDIENTS:

- 1/2 cup cooked quinoa
- 1/4 cup mixed berries (strawberries, blueberries, raspberries)
- 2 tablespoons chopped almonds
- 1 tablepoon honey
- 1/4 teaspoon cinnamon

INSTRUCTIONS:

1. In a bowl, combine cooked quinoa, mixed berries, chopped almonds, honey, and cinnamon.
2. Stir well to combine.
3. Serve immediately.

PREP TIME: 5 MINUTES

Nutritional Values (per serving):

- Calories: 220

- Protein: 6g
- Carbohydrates: 35g
- Fat: 6g

3. Greek Yogurt and Fruit Parfait:

INGREDIENTS:
- 1/2 cup low-fat Greek yogurt
- 1/4 cup diced mango
- 1/4 cup diced pineapple
- 2 tablespoons granola

INSTRUCTIONS:

1. In a glass, layer Greek yogurt, diced mango, diced pineapple, and granola.

2. Repeat layers as desired.

3. Serve chilled.

PREP TIME: 5 MINUTES

Nutritional Values (per serving):
- Calories: 180
- Protein: 10g
- Carbohydrates: 30g
- Fat: 3g

4. Spinach and Feta Breakfast Wrap:

INGREDIENTS:

- 1 whole grain tortilla
- 2 large eggs, scrambled
- 1/4 cup chopped spinach
- 2 tablespoons crumbled feta cheese

INSTRUCTIONS:

1. Heat the tortilla in a skillet over medium heat until warm.

2. Fill the tortilla with scrambled eggs, chopped spinach, and crumbled feta cheese.

3. Roll up the tortilla and serve.

PREP TIME: 10 MINUTES

Nutritional Values (per serving):

- Calories: 280
- Protein: 18g
- Carbohydrates: 20g
- Fat: 14g

5. Peanut Butter Banana Smoothie:

INGREDIENTS:
- 1 ripe banana
- 1 tablespoon natural peanut butter
- 1/2 cup low-fat milk or almond milk
- 1/4 cup plain Greek yogurt
- 1/2 cup ice cubes

INSTRUCTIONS:

1. In a blender, combine banana, peanut butter, milk, Greek yogurt, and ice cubes.

2. Blend until smooth.

3. Pour into a glass and serve immediately.

PREP TIME: 5 MINUTES

Nutritional Values (per serving):
- Calories: 250
- Protein: 13g
- Carbohydrates: 30g
- Fat: 10g

6. Whole Wheat Pancakes with Berries:

INGREDIENTS:

- 1/2 cup whole wheat flour
- 1/2 teaspoon baking powder
- 1/4 teaspoon cinnamon
- 1/2 cup low-fat milk
- 1 large egg
- 1/2 cup mixed berries (strawberries, blueberries)
- 1 tablespoon maple syrup

INSTRUCTIONS:

1. In a bowl, whisk together whole wheat flour, baking powder, and cinnamon.

2. In another bowl, whisk together milk and egg.

3. Gradually add the wet ingredients to the dry ingredients and stir until smooth.

4. Heat a skillet over medium heat and lightly grease with cooking spray.

5. Pour the pancake batter onto the skillet and cook until bubbles form on the surface. Flip and cook until golden brown.

6. Serve pancakes topped with mixed berries and maple syrup.

PREP TIME: 15 MINUTES

Nutritional Values (per serving):

- Calories: 280
- Protein: 10g
- Carbohydrates: 45g
- Fat: 6g

7. Avocado Toast with Poached Egg:

INGREDIENTS:

- 1 slice whole grain bread, toasted
- 1/2 ripe avocado, mashed
- 1 large egg, poached
- Salt and pepper to taste

INSTRUCTIONS:

1. Spread mashed avocado onto the toasted whole grain bread.
2. Top with a poached egg.
3. Season with salt and pepper to taste.

PREP TIME: 10 MINUTES

Nutritional Values (per serving):

- Calories: 250
- Protein: 12g
- Carbohydrates: 20g

- Fat: 14g

8. Overnight Chia Seed Pudding:

INGREDIENTS:

- 2 tablespoons chia seeds
- 1/2 cup low-fat milk or almond milk
- 1/2 teaspoon vanilla extract
- 1 tablespoon honey
- Fresh berries for topping

INSTRUCTIONS:

1. In a jar or bowl, combine chia seeds, milk, vanilla extract, and honey.

2. Stir well to combine.

3. Cover and refrigerate overnight.

4. In the morning, top with fresh berries before serving.

PREP TIME: 5 MINUTES (+ OVERNIGHT CHILLING)

Nutritional Values (per serving):

- Calories: 200
- Protein: 6g
- Carbohydrates: 20g

- Fat: 10g

9. Turkey and Veggie Breakfast Burrito:

INGREDIENTS:
- 1 whole grain tortilla
- 2 large eggs, scrambled
- 2 slices turkey bacon, cooked and chopped
- 1/4 cup diced bell peppers
- 1/4 cup diced onions
- Salsa for topping

INSTRUCTIONS:

1. Heat the tortilla in a skillet over medium heat until warm.

2. Fill the tortilla with scrambled eggs, chopped turkey bacon, diced bell peppers, and diced onions.

3. Roll up the tortilla and serve with salsa on top.

PREP TIME: 10 MINUTES

Nutritional Values (per serving):
- Calories: 280
- Protein: 18g
- Carbohydrates: 20g

- Fat: 14g

10. Almond Butter and Banana Toast:

INGREDIENTS:

- 1 slice whole grain bread, toasted
- 1 tablespoon almond butter
- 1/2 banana, sliced
- 1 teaspoon honey (optional)

INSTRUCTIONS:

1. Spread almond butter onto the toasted whole grain bread.

2. Top with sliced banana.

3. Drizzle with honey if desired.

PREP TIME: 5 MINUTES

Nutritional Values (per serving):

- Calories: 250
- Protein: 8g
- Carbohydrates: 30g
- Fat: 12g

CHAPTER 6: LUNCH RECIPES

1. Grilled Chicken Salad:

INGREDIENTS:

- 4 oz grilled chicken breast, sliced
- Mixed salad greens
- Cherry tomatoes, halved
- Cucumber, sliced
- Red onion, thinly sliced
- Balsamic vinaigrette dressing (low-sodium)

INSTRUCTIONS:

1. Arrange mixed salad greens on a plate.

2. Top with grilled chicken slices, cherry tomatoes, cucumber slices, and red onion.

3. Drizzle with balsamic vinaigrette dressing.

PREP TIME: 15 MINUTES

Nutritional Values (per serving):

- Calories: 250
- Protein: 25g
- Carbohydrates: 10g
- Fat: 12g

2. Quinoa and Black Bean Salad:

INGREDIENTS:

- 1/2 cup cooked quinoa
- 1/2 cup black beans, drained and rinsed
- Diced bell peppers (any color)
- Diced tomatoes
- Chopped cilantro
- Lime juice
- Olive oil
- Salt and pepper to taste

INSTRUCTIONS:

1. In a bowl, combine cooked quinoa, black beans, diced bell peppers, diced tomatoes, and chopped cilantro.
2. Drizzle with lime juice and olive oil.
3. Season with salt and pepper to taste.

PREP TIME: 15 MINUTES

Nutritional Values (per serving):

- Calories: 280
- Protein: 10g
- Carbohydrates: 40g
- Fat: 8g

3. Tuna Salad Lettuce Wraps:

INGREDIENTS:
- 1 can (5 oz) tuna in water, drained
- Greek yogurt (plain, low-fat)
- Diced celery
- Diced red onion
- Dijon mustard
- Lettuce leaves (such as romaine or butterhead)

INSTRUCTIONS:

1. In a bowl, mix together drained tuna, Greek yogurt, diced celery, diced red onion, and Dijon mustard.

2. Spoon the tuna salad mixture onto lettuce leaves.

3. Roll up the lettuce leaves and serve.

PREP TIME: 10 MINUTES

Nutritional Values (per serving):
- Calories: 180
- Protein: 20g
- Carbohydrates: 5g
- Fat: 8g

4. Vegetable Stir-Fry with Brown Rice:

INGREDIENTS:

- Mixed vegetables (bell peppers, broccoli, carrots, snap peas)
- Low-sodium soy sauce
- Minced garlic
- Cooked brown rice
- Sesame oil
- Green onions, chopped (for garnish)

INSTRUCTIONS:

1. In a skillet, heat sesame oil over medium heat.
2. Add minced garlic and stir-fry for 1 minute.
3. Add mixed vegetables and stir-fry until tender-crisp.
4. Stir in low-sodium soy sauce and cooked brown rice.
5. Cook until heated through.
6. Garnish with chopped green onions before serving.

PREP TIME: 20 MINUTES

Nutritional Values (per serving):

- Calories: 300
- Protein: 8g
- Carbohydrates: 50g
- Fat: 6g

5. Turkey and Avocado Wrap:

INGREDIENTS:

- Whole grain tortilla
- Sliced turkey breast
- Avocado slices
- Spinach leaves
- Diced tomatoes
- Hummus (optional)

INSTRUCTIONS:

1. Lay a whole grain tortilla flat.

2. Layer sliced turkey breast, avocado slices, spinach leaves, and diced tomatoes on the tortilla.

3. Spread hummus (if using) on top.

4. Roll up the tortilla and slice in half.

PREP TIME: 10 MINUTES

Nutritional Values (per serving):

- Calories: 280
- Protein: 18g
- Carbohydrates: 30g
- Fat: 12g

6. Lentil Soup:

INGREDIENTS:

- 1 cup dried lentils
- Vegetable broth (low-sodium)
- Diced carrots
- Diced celery
- Diced onions
- Minced garlic
- Bay leaf
- Chopped parsley (for garnish)

INSTRUCTIONS:

1. Rinse lentils under cold water and drain.

2. In a large pot, combine lentils, vegetable broth, diced carrots, diced celery, diced onions, minced garlic, and bay leaf.

3. Bring to a boil, then reduce heat and simmer until lentils are tender.

4. Remove bay leaf before serving.

5. Garnish with chopped parsley.

PREP TIME: 15 MINUTES

Nutritional Values (per serving):

- Calories: 250
- Protein: 18g
- Carbohydrates: 40g
- Fat: 2g

7. Grilled Veggie Wrap:

INGREDIENTS:

- Whole grain tortilla
- Grilled vegetables (zucchini, bell peppers, eggplant)
- Hummus
- Baby spinach leaves
- Sliced tomatoes

INSTRUCTIONS:

1. Lay a whole grain tortilla flat.
2. Spread hummus evenly over the tortilla.
3. Layer grilled vegetables, baby spinach leaves, and sliced tomatoes on top.
4. Roll up the tortilla and slice in half.

PREP TIME: 15 MINUTES

Nutritional Values (per serving):

- Calories: 220

- Protein: 8g
- Carbohydrates: 30g
- Fat: 8g

8. Chicken and Vegetable Stir-Fry:

INGREDIENTS:

- 4 oz boneless, skinless chicken breast, sliced
- Mixed vegetables (broccoli, bell peppers, snap peas, carrots)
- Low-sodium stir-fry sauce
- Cooked brown rice
- Sesame oil
- Green onions, chopped (for garnish)

INSTRUCTIONS:

1. In a skillet, heat sesame oil over medium heat.
2. Add sliced chicken breast and stir-fry until cooked through.
3. Add mixed vegetables and stir-fry until tender-crisp.
4. Stir in low-sodium stir-fry sauce and cook until heated through.
5. Serve over cooked brown rice.

6. Garnish with chopped green onions.

PREP TIME: 20 MINUTES

Nutritional Values (per serving):
- Calories: 300
- Protein: 25g
- Carbohydrates: 35g
- Fat: 8g

9. Mediterranean Chickpea Salad:

INGREDIENTS:
- 1 can (15 oz) chickpeas (garbanzo beans), drained and rinsed
- Diced cucumber
- Diced tomatoes
- Chopped red onion
- Kalamata olives, pitted and halved
- Crumbled feta cheese
- Lemon juice
- Extra virgin olive oil
- Chopped parsley (for garnish)

INSTRUCTIONS:

1. In a large bowl, combine chickpeas, diced cucumber, diced tomatoes, chopped red onion, halved Kalamata olives, and crumbled feta cheese.

2. Drizzle with lemon juice and extra virgin olive oil.

3. Toss to combine.

4. Garnish with chopped parsley before serving.

PREP TIME: 15 MINUTES

Nutritional Values (per serving):

- Calories: 280
- Protein: 12g
- Carbohydrates: 35g
- Fat: 10g

10. Egg Salad Lettuce Wraps:

INGREDIENTS:

- 4 hard-boiled eggs, chopped
- Greek yogurt (plain, low-fat)
- Diced celery
- Diced red onion
- Dijon mustard
- Lettuce leaves (such as romaine or butterhead)

INSTRUCTIONS:

1. In a bowl, mix together chopped hard-boiled eggs, Greek yogurt, diced celery, diced red onion, and Dijon mustard.

2. Spoon the egg salad mixture onto lettuce leaves.

3. Roll up the lettuce leaves and serve.

PREP TIME: 10 MINUTES

Nutritional Values (per serving):

- Calories: 200
- Protein: 14g
- Carbohydrates: 5g
- Fat: 12g

CHAPTER 7: DINNER RECIPES

1. Baked Salmon with Roasted Vegetables:

Ingredients:
- 4 oz salmon fillet
- Mixed vegetables (such as broccoli, bell peppers, carrots)
- Olive oil
- Lemon juice
- Garlic powder
- Salt and pepper to taste

INSTRUCTIONS:

1. Preheat the oven to 400°F (200°C).

2. Place salmon fillet on a baking sheet lined with parchment paper.

3. Arrange mixed vegetables around the salmon.

4. Drizzle olive oil and lemon juice over the salmon and vegetables.

5. Season with garlic powder, salt, and pepper.

6. Bake for 15-20 minutes or until salmon is cooked through and vegetables are tender.

PREP TIME: 20 MINUTES

Nutritional Values (per serving):
- Calories: 300
- Protein: 25g
- Carbohydrates: 15g
- Fat: 15g

2. Turkey Chili:

INGREDIENTS:
- 1 lb lean ground turkey
- Diced onions
- Diced bell peppers
- Diced tomatoes
- Kidney beans (canned, drained and rinsed)
- Low-sodium tomato sauce
- Chili powder
- Cumin
- Garlic powder
- Salt and pepper to taste

INSTRUCTIONS:

1. In a large pot, cook ground turkey over medium heat until browned.

2. Add diced onions and bell peppers, and cook until softened.

3. Stir in diced tomatoes, kidney beans, and tomato sauce.

4. Season with chili powder, cumin, garlic powder, salt, and pepper.

5. Simmer for 20-30 minutes, stirring occasionally.

PREP TIME: 30 MINUTES

Nutritional Values (per serving):

- Calories: 250
- Protein: 20g
- Carbohydrates: 25g
- Fat: 8g

3. Lemon Herb Grilled Chicken:

INGREDIENTS:

- 4 oz chicken breast
- Lemon juice
- Olive oil
- Minced garlic

- Chopped fresh herbs (such as parsley, thyme, rosemary)
- Salt and pepper to taste

INSTRUCTIONS:

1. In a bowl, mix together lemon juice, olive oil, minced garlic, chopped herbs, salt, and pepper.

2. Marinate chicken breast in the mixture for 30 minutes to 1 hour.

3. Preheat grill to medium-high heat.

4. Grill chicken breast for 6-8 minutes per side or until cooked through.

PREP TIME: 40 MINUTES (INCLUDING MARINATING TIME)

Nutritional Values (per serving):

- Calories: 200
- Protein: 25g
- Carbohydrates: 1g
- Fat: 10g

4. Vegetable Stir-Fry with Tofu:

INGREDIENTS:

- 4 oz firm tofu, cubed

- Mixed vegetables (such as broccoli, bell peppers, snap peas, carrots)
- Low-sodium stir-fry sauce
- Cooked brown rice
- Sesame oil
- Green onions, chopped (for garnish)

INSTRUCTIONS:

1. In a skillet, heat sesame oil over medium heat.
2. Add cubed tofu and stir-fry until lightly browned.
3. Add mixed vegetables and stir-fry until tender-crisp.
4. Stir in low-sodium stir-fry sauce and cook until heated through.
5. Serve over cooked brown rice.
6. Garnish with chopped green onions.

PREP TIME: 20 MINUTES

Nutritional Values (per serving):

- Calories: 300
- Protein: 15g
- Carbohydrates: 35g
- Fat: 10g

5. Shrimp and Vegetable Skewers:

INGREDIENTS:

- 4 oz shrimp, peeled and deveined
- Mixed vegetables (such as cherry tomatoes, bell peppers, zucchini)
- Olive oil
- Lemon juice
- Garlic powder
- Salt and pepper to taste

INSTRUCTIONS:

1. Preheat grill to medium-high heat.
2. Thread shrimp and mixed vegetables onto skewers.
3. Drizzle olive oil and lemon juice over skewers.
4. Season with garlic powder, salt, and pepper.
5. Grill skewers for 2-3 minutes per side or until shrimp is pink and vegetables are tender.

PREP TIME: 20 MINUTES

Nutritional Values (per serving):

- Calories: 200
- Protein: 20g
- Carbohydrates: 10g
- Fat: 8g

6. Baked Cod with Herbed Quinoa:

INGREDIENTS:

- 4 oz cod fillet
- Lemon juice
- Olive oil
- Chopped fresh herbs (such as parsley, dill, chives)
- Cooked quinoa
- Steamed green beans

INSTRUCTIONS:

1. Preheat the oven to 400°F (200°C).
2. Place cod fillet on a baking sheet lined with parchment paper.
3. Drizzle with lemon juice and olive oil.
4. Sprinkle chopped fresh herbs over the cod.
5. Bake for 15-20 minutes or until cod is cooked through.
6. Serve with cooked quinoa and steamed green beans.

PREP TIME: 25 MINUTES

Nutritional Values (per serving):

- Calories: 250
- Protein: 25g

- Carbohydrates: 20g
- Fat: 8g

7. Beef and Vegetable Stir-Fry:

INGREDIENTS:

- 4 oz lean beef strips (such as sirloin or flank steak)
- Mixed vegetables (such as broccoli, bell peppers, snap peas, carrots)
- Low-sodium stir-fry sauce
- Cooked brown rice
- Sesame oil
- Green onions, chopped (for garnish)

INSTRUCTIONS:

1. In a skillet, heat sesame oil over medium heat.
2. Add beef strips and stir-fry until browned.
3. Add mixed vegetables and stir-fry until tender-crisp.
4. Stir in low-sodium stir-fry sauce and cook until heated through.
5. Serve over cooked brown rice.
6. Garnish with chopped green onions.

PREP TIME: 20 MINUTES

Nutritional Values (per serving):

- Calories: 300
- Protein: 20g
- Carbohydrates: 35g
- Fat: 10g

8. Stuffed Bell Peppers:

INGREDIENTS:

- Bell peppers (any color), halved and seeded
- Lean ground turkey or chicken
- Cooked quinoa
- Diced tomatoes
- Diced onions
- Minced garlic
- Italian seasoning
- Low-sodium tomato sauce

INSTRUCTIONS:

1. Preheat the oven to 375°F (190°C).

2. In a skillet, cook ground turkey or chicken until browned.

3. Add cooked quinoa, diced tomatoes, diced onions, minced garlic, Italian seasoning, and tomato sauce to the skillet. Stir to combine.

4. Spoon the mixture into halved bell peppers.

5. Place stuffed bell peppers in a baking dish and cover with foil.

6. Bake for 30-35 minutes or until peppers are tender.

PREP TIME: 30 MINUTES

Nutritional Values (per serving):

- Calories: 280
- Protein: 25g
- Carbohydrates: 25g
- Fat: 10g

9. Veggie and Tofu Stir-Fry:

INGREDIENTS:

- 4 oz firm tofu, cubed
- Mixed vegetables (such as broccoli, bell peppers, snap peas, carrots)
- Low-sodium stir-fry sauce
- Cooked quinoa or brown rice

- Sesame oil
- Green onions, chopped (for garnish)

INSTRUCTIONS:

1. In a skillet, heat sesame oil over medium heat.
2. Add cubed tofu and stir-fry until lightly browned.
3. Add mixed vegetables and stir-fry until tender-crisp.
4. Stir in low-sodium stir-fry sauce and cook until heated through.
5. Serve over cooked quinoa or brown rice.
6. Garnish with chopped green onions.

PREP TIME: 20 MINUTES

Nutritional Values (per serving):

- Calories: 280
- Protein: 15g
- Carbohydrates: 35g
- Fat: 10g

10. Lemon Garlic Shrimp Pasta:

INGREDIENTS:

- 4 oz whole wheat pasta
- 4 oz shrimp, peeled and deveined
- Olive oil

- Minced garlic
- Lemon zest
- Lemon juice
- Chopped parsley
- Salt and pepper to taste

INSTRUCTIONS:

1. Cook whole wheat pasta according to package instructions. Drain and set aside.

2. In a skillet, heat olive oil over medium heat.

3. Add minced garlic and cook until fragrant.

4. Add shrimp to the skillet and cook until pink and cooked through.

5. Stir in lemon zest and lemon juice.

6. Add cooked pasta to the skillet and toss to coat.

7. Season with chopped parsley, salt, and pepper.

8. Serve immediately.

PREP TIME: 25 MINUTES

Nutritional Values (per serving):

- Calories: 300
- Protein: 20g
- Carbohydrates: 35g
- Fat: 8g

CHAPTER 7: SNACK AND APPETIZER IDEAS

1. Hummus and Veggie Sticks:

INGREDIENTS:

- 1 can (15 oz) chickpeas (garbanzo beans), drained and rinsed
- Lemon juice
- Olive oil
- Minced garlic
- Tahini (optional)
- Carrot sticks, cucumber slices, bell pepper strips (for dipping)

INSTRUCTIONS:

1. In a food processor, combine chickpeas, lemon juice, olive oil, minced garlic, and tahini (if using).

2. Blend until smooth and creamy, adding water as needed to achieve desired consistency.

3. Serve hummus with vegetable sticks for dipping.

PREP TIME: 10 MINUTES

Nutritional Values (per serving):

- Calories: 100

- Protein: 4g
- Carbohydrates: 12g
- Fat: 5g

2. Greek Yogurt Dip with Whole Grain Crackers:

INGREDIENTS:
- Plain Greek yogurt (low-fat)
- Lemon juice
- Chopped fresh dill
- Minced garlic
- Salt and pepper to taste
- Whole grain crackers

INSTRUCTIONS:

1. In a bowl, mix together Greek yogurt, lemon juice, chopped fresh dill, minced garlic, salt, and pepper.

2. Stir until well combined.

3. Serve with whole grain crackers for dipping.

PREP TIME: 5 MINUTES

Nutritional Values (per serving):
- Calories: 80

- Protein: 6g
- Carbohydrates: 10g
- Fat: 2g

3. Caprese Skewers:

INGREDIENTS:

- Cherry tomatoes
- Fresh mozzarella balls
- Fresh basil leaves
- Balsamic glaze (optional)

INSTRUCTIONS:

1. Thread cherry tomatoes, fresh mozzarella balls, and fresh basil leaves onto skewers.
2. Drizzle with balsamic glaze if desired.
3. Serve immediately.

PREP TIME: 10 MINUTES

Nutritional Values (per serving):

- Calories: 100
- Protein: 6g
- Carbohydrates: 4g
- Fat: 6g

4. Cucumber and Cream Cheese Roll-Ups:

INGREDIENTS:

- English cucumber
- Low-fat cream cheese
- Smoked salmon slices (optional)

INSTRUCTIONS:

1. Using a vegetable peeler, slice the cucumber lengthwise into thin strips.

2. Spread a thin layer of low-fat cream cheese on each cucumber strip.

3. Place a slice of smoked salmon (if using) on top of the cream cheese.

4. Roll up the cucumber strip and secure with a toothpick.

PREP TIME: 10 MINUTES

Nutritional Values (per serving):

- Calories: 50
- Protein: 2g
- Carbohydrates: 2g
- Fat: 4g

5. Apple Slices with Almond Butter:

INGREDIENTS:
- Apple, sliced
- Almond butter (unsweetened)

INSTRUCTIONS:
1. Spread almond butter onto apple slices.
2. Serve immediately.

PREP TIME: 5 MINUTES

Nutritional Values (per serving):
- Calories: 120
- Protein: 3g
- Carbohydrates: 15g
- Fat: 7g

6. Cottage Cheese with Pineapple:

INGREDIENTS:
- Low-fat cottage cheese
- Fresh pineapple chunks

INSTRUCTIONS:
1. Serve low-fat cottage cheese with fresh pineapple chunks.

2. Enjoy as a refreshing snack.

PREP TIME: 5 MINUTES

Nutritional Values (per serving):
- Calories: 120
- Protein: 14g
- Carbohydrates: 15g
- Fat: 2g

7. Edamame Hummus with Whole Grain Pita Chips:

INGREDIENTS:
- 1 cup shelled edamame (frozen, thawed)
- Lemon juice
- Olive oil
- Minced garlic
- Tahini (optional)
- Whole grain pita chips

INSTRUCTIONS:

1. In a food processor, combine shelled edamame, lemon juice, olive oil, minced garlic, and tahini (if using).

2. Blend until smooth and creamy, adding water as needed to achieve desired consistency.

3. Serve edamame hummus with whole grain pita chips for dipping.

PREP TIME: 10 MINUTES

Nutritional Values (per serving):
- Calories: 100
- Protein: 6g
- Carbohydrates: 10g
- Fat: 4g

8. Avocado Salsa with Baked Tortilla Chips:

INGREDIENTS:
- Ripe avocado, diced
- Diced tomatoes
- Diced red onion
- Chopped cilantro
- Lime juice
- Salt and pepper to taste
- Whole grain tortillas

INSTRUCTIONS:

1. In a bowl, combine diced avocado, diced tomatoes, diced red onion, chopped cilantro, lime juice, salt, and pepper.

2. Mix gently until well combined.

3. Serve avocado salsa with baked whole grain tortilla chips.

PREP TIME: 15 MINUTES

Nutritional Values (per serving):

- Calories: 120
- Protein: 2g
- Carbohydrates: 15g
- Fat: 6g

9. Roasted Chickpeas:

INGREDIENTS:

- 1 can (15 oz) chickpeas (garbanzo beans), drained and rinsed
- Olive oil
- Salt and pepper
- Optional seasonings (such as paprika, cumin, garlic powder)

INSTRUCTIONS:

1. Preheat the oven to 400°F (200°C).

2. Pat dry the chickpeas with a paper towel to remove excess moisture.

3. In a bowl, toss chickpeas with olive oil, salt, pepper, and optional seasonings.

4. Spread chickpeas in a single layer on a baking sheet lined with parchment paper.

5. Bake for 20-30 minutes or until crispy, shaking the pan occasionally.

6. Let cool before serving.

PREP TIME: 5 MINUTES (PLUS BAKING TIME)
Nutritional Values (per serving):
- Calories: 100
- Protein: 4g
- Carbohydrates: 15g
- Fat: 3g

10. Stuffed Mini Bell Peppers:
INGREDIENTS:
- Mini bell peppers, halved and seeded
- Low-fat cream cheese
- Chopped fresh chives

- Diced tomatoes
- Salt and pepper to taste

INSTRUCTIONS:

1. In a bowl, mix together low-fat cream cheese, chopped fresh chives, diced tomatoes, salt, and pepper.

2. Spoon the cream cheese mixture into halved mini bell peppers.

3. Serve immediately or refrigerate until ready to serve.

PREP TIME: 15 MINUTES

Nutritional Values (per serving):

- Calories: 80
- Protein: 2g
- Carbohydrates: 10g
- Fat: 4g

CHAPTER 8: DESSERTS RECIPES

1. Fruit Salad with Honey-Lime Dressing:

INGREDIENTS:
- Mixed fruits (such as berries, melon, grapes, pineapple)
- Fresh lime juice
- Honey

INSTRUCTIONS:

1. Wash and chop the mixed fruits as needed.

2. In a bowl, whisk together fresh lime juice and honey to make the dressing.

3. Pour the dressing over the mixed fruits and toss gently to coat.

4. Serve immediately or chill before serving.

PREP TIME: 10 MINUTES

Nutritional Values (per serving):
- Calories: 80
- Protein: 1g
- Carbohydrates: 20g
- Fat: 0g

2. Greek Yogurt Parfait with Berries and Granola:

INGREDIENTS:

- Plain Greek yogurt (low-fat)
- Mixed berries (such as strawberries, blueberries, raspberries)
- Low-sugar granola

INSTRUCTIONS:

1. In a glass or bowl, layer Greek yogurt, mixed berries, and low-sugar granola.
2. Repeat the layers as desired.
3. Serve immediately.

PREP TIME: 5 MINUTES

Nutritional Values (per serving):

- Calories: 150
- Protein: 10g
- Carbohydrates: 25g
- Fat: 3g

3. Baked Apples with Cinnamon and Walnuts:

INGREDIENTS:

- Apples, cored
- Ground cinnamon
- Chopped walnuts
- Honey (optional)

INSTRUCTIONS:

1. Preheat the oven to 375°F (190°C).
2. Place cored apples in a baking dish.
3. Sprinkle ground cinnamon and chopped walnuts over the apples.
4. Drizzle with honey if desired.
5. Bake for 20-25 minutes or until apples are tender.
6. Serve warm.

PREP TIME: 10 MINUTES

Nutritional Values (per serving):

- Calories: 120
- Protein: 2g
- Carbohydrates: 20g
- Fat: 5g

4. Frozen Yogurt Bark with Mixed Nuts and Berries:

INGREDIENTS:
- Plain Greek yogurt (low-fat)
- Mixed nuts (such as almonds, walnuts, pistachios)
- Mixed berries (such as strawberries, blueberries, raspberries)
- Honey (optional)

INSTRUCTIONS:

1. Line a baking sheet with parchment paper.
2. Spread Greek yogurt evenly onto the parchment paper.
3. Sprinkle mixed nuts and mixed berries over the yogurt.
4. Drizzle with honey if desired.
5. Freeze for 2-3 hours or until firm.
6. Break into pieces before serving.

PREP TIME: 10 MINUTES (PLUS FREEZING TIME)

Nutritional Values (per serving):
- Calories: 150
- Protein: 8g
- Carbohydrates: 15g

- Fat: 7g

5. Chocolate Avocado Mousse:

INGREDIENTS:

- Ripe avocados
- Unsweetened cocoa powder
- Honey or maple syrup
- Vanilla extract

INSTRUCTIONS:

1. Scoop the flesh of ripe avocados into a blender or food processor.

2. Add unsweetened cocoa powder, honey or maple syrup, and vanilla extract.

3. Blend until smooth and creamy.

4. Divide into serving dishes and chill before serving.

PREP TIME: 10 MINUTES

Nutritional Values (per serving):

- Calories: 150
- Protein: 2g
- Carbohydrates: 10g
- Fat: 12g

6. Banana Oatmeal Cookies:

INGREDIENTS:

- Ripe bananas, mashed
- Rolled oats
- Cinnamon
- Chopped nuts (such as walnuts or almonds)
- Raisins or dried cranberries (optional)

INSTRUCTIONS:

1. Preheat the oven to 350°F (175°C) and line a baking sheet with parchment paper.

2. In a bowl, mix together mashed bananas, rolled oats, cinnamon, chopped nuts, and raisins or dried cranberries (if using).

3. Drop spoonfuls of the mixture onto the prepared baking sheet.

4. Flatten each cookie with the back of a spoon.

5. Bake for 15-20 minutes or until golden brown.

6. Let cool before serving.

PREP TIME: 10 MINUTES

Nutritional Values (per serving, approximate, based on 1 cookie):

- Calories: 60
- Protein: 1g
- Carbohydrates: 10g
- Fat: 2g

7. Chia Seed Pudding with Fresh Fruit:
INGREDIENTS:

Chia seeds

Unsweetened almond milk

Honey or maple syrup

Fresh fruit (such as berries, sliced kiwi, mango)

INSTRUCTIONS:

1. In a bowl or jar, mix together chia seeds, unsweetened almond milk, and honey or maple syrup.

2. Stir well and refrigerate for at least 2 hours or overnight, stirring occasionally until thickened.

3. Serve chilled with fresh fruit on top.

PREP TIME: 5 MINUTES (PLUS CHILLING TIME)

Nutritional Values (per serving):

- Calories: 120
- Protein: 3g
- Carbohydrates: 15g

- Fat: 5g

8. Strawberry Banana Smoothie:

INGREDIENTS:

- Fresh or frozen strawberries
- Ripe banana
- Plain Greek yogurt (low-fat)
- Unsweetened almond milk
- Honey or maple syrup (optional)

INSTRUCTIONS:

1. In a blender, combine strawberries, banana, Greek yogurt, unsweetened almond milk, and honey or maple syrup (if using).

2. Blend until smooth and creamy.

3. Pour into glasses and serve immediately.

PREP TIME: 5 MINUTES

Nutritional Values (per serving):

- Calories: 150
- Protein: 8g
- Carbohydrates: 25g
- Fat: 2g

9. Almond Flour Blueberry Muffins:

INGREDIENTS:

- Almond flour
- Baking powder
- Salt
- Eggs
- Unsweetened applesauce
- Honey or maple syrup
- Vanilla extract
- Fresh or frozen blueberries

INSTRUCTIONS:

1. Preheat the oven to 350°F (175°C) and line a muffin tin with paper liners.

2. In a bowl, whisk together almond flour, baking powder, and salt.

3. In another bowl, mix together eggs, unsweetened applesauce, honey or maple syrup, and vanilla extract.

4. Gradually add the wet ingredients to the dry ingredients and mix until well combined.

5. Gently fold in the blueberries.

6. Divide the batter evenly among the muffin cups.

7. Bake for 20-25 minutes or until a toothpick inserted into the center comes out clean.

8. Let cool before serving.

PREP TIME: 15 MINUTES

Nutritional Values (per serving, approximate, based on 1 muffin):

- Calories: 120
- Protein: 4g
- Carbohydrates: 10g
- Fat: 8g

10. Coconut Mango Rice Pudding:

INGREDIENTS:

- Cooked brown rice
- Coconut milk (unsweetened)
- Diced mango
- Unsweetened shredded coconut
- Honey or maple syrup (optional)

INSTRUCTIONS:

1. In a saucepan, combine cooked brown rice and coconut milk.

2. Cook over medium heat, stirring occasionally, until thickened.

3. Stir in diced mango and unsweetened shredded coconut.

4. Sweeten with honey or maple syrup if desired.

5. Cook for an additional 2-3 minutes.

6. Serve warm or chilled.

PREP TIME: 15 MINUTES

Nutritional Values (per serving):
- Calories: 150
- Protein: 3g
- Carbohydrates: 20g
- Fat: 7g

CHAPTER 9: SMOOTHIE RECIPES

1. Green Power Smoothie:

INGREDIENTS:

- Spinach leaves
- Kale leaves
- Frozen banana
- Unsweetened almond milk
- Greek yogurt (low-fat)
- Honey or maple syrup (optional)

INSTRUCTIONS:

1. Place spinach leaves, kale leaves, frozen banana, almond milk, and Greek yogurt in a blender.
2. Blend until smooth and creamy.
3. Sweeten with honey or maple syrup if desired.
4. Serve immediately.

PREP TIME: 5 MINUTES

Nutritional Values (per serving):

- Calories: 150
- Protein: 8g
- Carbohydrates: 25g
- Fat: 2g

2. Berry Blast Smoothie:

INGREDIENTS:

- Mixed berries (such as strawberries, blueberries, raspberries)
- Frozen banana
- Plain Greek yogurt (low-fat)
- Unsweetened almond milk

INSTRUCTIONS:

1. Combine mixed berries, frozen banana, Greek yogurt, and almond milk in a blender.
2. Blend until smooth and creamy.
3. Serve immediately.

PREP TIME: 5 MINUTES

Nutritional Values (per serving):

- Calories: 120
- Protein: 6g
- Carbohydrates: 20g
- Fat: 2g

3. Tropical Paradise Smoothie:

INGREDIENTS:
- Pineapple chunks (fresh or frozen)
- Mango chunks (fresh or frozen)
- Banana
- Coconut milk (unsweetened)
- Greek yogurt (low-fat)

INSTRUCTIONS:

1. Place pineapple chunks, mango chunks, banana, coconut milk, and Greek yogurt in a blender.
2. Blend until smooth and creamy.
3. Serve immediately.

PREP TIME: 5 MINUTES

Nutritional Values (per serving):
- Calories: 150
- Protein: 6g
- Carbohydrates: 25g
- Fat: 3g

4. Peanut Butter Banana Smoothie:

INGREDIENTS:

- Ripe banana
- Natural peanut butter
- Unsweetened almond milk
- Greek yogurt (low-fat)
- Honey or maple syrup (optional)

INSTRUCTIONS:

1. Combine ripe banana, peanut butter, almond milk, Greek yogurt, and honey or maple syrup (if using) in a blender.

2. Blend until smooth and creamy.

3. Serve immediately.

PREP TIME: 5 MINUTES

Nutritional Values (per serving):

- Calories: 200
- Protein: 10g
- Carbohydrates: 25g
- Fat: 8g

5. Creamy Avocado Smoothie:

INGREDIENTS:

- Ripe avocado

- Banana
- Unsweetened almond milk
- Greek yogurt (low-fat)
- Honey or maple syrup (optional)

INSTRUCTIONS:

1. Blend ripe avocado, banana, almond milk, Greek yogurt, and honey or maple syrup (if using) until smooth and creamy.

2. Serve immediately.

PREP TIME: 5 MINUTES

Nutritional Values (per serving):
- Calories: 180
- Protein: 6g
- Carbohydrates: 25g
- Fat: 8g

6. Mixed Berry and Spinach Smoothie:

INGREDIENTS:

- Mixed berries (such as strawberries, blueberries, raspberries)
- Spinach leaves

- Frozen banana
- Unsweetened almond milk

INSTRUCTIONS:

1. Blend mixed berries, spinach leaves, frozen banana, and almond milk until smooth and creamy.

2. Serve immediately.

PREP TIME: 5 MINUTES

Nutritional Values (per serving):
- Calories: 120
- Protein: 4g
- Carbohydrates: 25g
- Fat: 2g

7. Mango Peach Smoothie:

INGREDIENTS:
- Mango chunks (fresh or frozen)
- Peach slices (fresh or frozen)
- Banana
- Unsweetened almond milk
- Greek yogurt (low-fat)

INSTRUCTIONS:

1. Blend mango chunks, peach slices, banana, almond milk, and Greek yogurt until smooth and creamy.

2. Serve immediately.

PREP TIME: 5 MINUTES

Nutritional Values (per serving):
- Calories: 150
- Protein: 6g
- Carbohydrates: 30g
- Fat: 2g

8. Blueberry Banana Smoothie:

INGREDIENTS:
- Blueberries (fresh or frozen)
- Banana
- Unsweetened almond milk
- Greek yogurt (low-fat)

INSTRUCTIONS:

1. Blend blueberries, banana, almond milk, and Greek yogurt until smooth and creamy.

2. Serve immediately.

PREP TIME: 5 MINUTES

Nutritional Values (per serving):

- Calories: 120
- Protein: 6g
- Carbohydrates: 25g
- Fat: 2g

9. Cherry Almond Smoothie:

INGREDIENTS:

- Cherries (pitted, fresh or frozen)
- Almond butter (unsweetened)
- Unsweetened almond milk
- Greek yogurt (low-fat)

INSTRUCTIONS:

1. Blend cherries, almond butter, almond milk, and Greek yogurt until smooth and creamy.
2. Serve immediately.

PREP TIME: 5 MINUTES

Nutritional Values (per serving):

- Calories: 150
- Protein: 8g
- Carbohydrates: 20g
- Fat: 5g

10. Raspberry Coconut Smoothie:

INGREDIENTS:

- Raspberries (fresh or frozen)
- Coconut milk (unsweetened)
- Banana
- Greek yogurt (low-fat)

INSTRUCTIONS:

1. Blend raspberries, coconut milk, banana, and Greek yogurt until smooth and creamy.

2. Serve immediately.

PREP TIME: 5 MINUTES

Nutritional Values (per serving):

- Calories: 150
- Protein: 6g
- Carbohydrates: 25g
- Fat: 3g

CHAPTER 10: FREQUENTLY ASKED QUESTIONS

Common Concerns and Queries about CKD and the DASH Diet

1. Can the DASH Diet benefit individuals with CKD?

- Yes, the DASH Diet can benefit individuals with CKD. It emphasizes fruits, vegetables, whole grains, lean proteins, and low-fat dairy, which are all components of a kidney-friendly diet. The DASH Diet also promotes reducing sodium intake, which is crucial for managing blood pressure and protecting kidney function.

2. Is the DASH Diet suitable for all stages of CKD?

- The DASH Diet can be adapted for all stages of CKD, but modifications may be necessary depending on individual kidney function and dietary restrictions. For example, those in later stages of CKD may need to further limit potassium, phosphorus, and protein intake. Consulting with a registered dietitian who specializes in kidney health can help tailor the DASH Diet to meet specific needs.

How does the DASH Diet help manage blood pressure in CKD?

- The DASH Diet is rich in fruits, vegetables, and low-fat dairy products, which provide essential nutrients like potassium, magnesium, and calcium. These nutrients help lower blood pressure by promoting vasodilation, reducing sodium retention, and improving overall vascular health. By following the DASH Diet, individuals with CKD can better control their blood pressure, reducing the risk of further kidney damage and cardiovascular complications.

Are there specific foods to avoid on the DASH Diet for CKD?

- While the DASH Diet emphasizes healthy food choices, individuals with CKD may need to limit certain foods to manage their condition effectively.

Foods high in sodium, potassium, phosphorus, and protein should be consumed in moderation or avoided, depending on individual dietary restrictions and kidney function. Examples include processed foods, canned soups, high-potassium fruits and vegetables, dairy products, and high-protein foods like red meat.

How can I incorporate the DASH Diet into my lifestyle if I have CKD?

- Incorporating the DASH Diet into your lifestyle with CKD involves making gradual changes to your eating habits. Start by increasing your intake of fruits, vegetables, whole grains, and lean proteins while reducing sodium, processed foods, and unhealthy fats. Meal planning and preparation can also help you adhere to the DASH Diet more easily. Consulting with a registered dietitian who specializes in kidney health can provide personalized guidance and support.

Can the DASH Diet help slow the progression of CKD?

- While the DASH Diet alone may not reverse CKD, it can help slow the progression of the disease by managing risk factors such as high blood pressure and cardiovascular disease. By promoting a healthy lifestyle and supporting overall kidney function, the DASH Diet plays a crucial role in preserving kidney health and improving quality of life for individuals with CKD.

What role does hydration play in CKD and the DASH Diet?

- Adequate hydration is essential for individuals with CKD to maintain kidney function and prevent complications such as dehydration and electrolyte imbalances. While the DASH Diet emphasizes consuming plenty of fruits and vegetables, which contribute to overall hydration, it's important to monitor fluid intake, especially for those with advanced CKD or fluid restrictions. Consulting with a healthcare professional can help determine individual fluid needs based on kidney function and medical history.

How can I manage protein intake on the DASH Diet for CKD?

- Managing protein intake on the DASH Diet for CKD involves choosing lean protein sources such as poultry, fish, tofu, and legumes while moderating portion sizes. Individuals with CKD may need to limit protein intake to reduce the burden on the kidneys, especially in later stages of the disease. A registered dietitian can provide personalized recommendations for protein intake based on individual nutritional needs and kidney function.

By addressing these common concerns and queries, individuals with CKD can better understand the role of the DASH Diet in managing their condition and improving overall health outcomes. It's essential to work closely with healthcare professionals and registered dietitians to develop a personalized dietary plan that meets individual needs and supports kidney health.

14-Day Meal Plan

DAY 1:

Breakfast: Greek Yogurt Parfait with Berries and Granola

Lunch: Caprese Salad with Grilled Chicken

Dinner: Baked Salmon with Roasted Asparagus and Quinoa

Snack: Apple Slices with Almond Butter

DAY 2:

Breakfast: Green Power Smoothie

Lunch: Hummus and Veggie Sticks

Dinner: Stuffed Bell Peppers with Ground Turkey and Brown Rice

Snack: Cottage Cheese with Pineapple

DAY 3:

Breakfast: Berry Blast Smoothie

Lunch: Greek Salad with Grilled Shrimp

Dinner: Chicken Stir-Fry with Mixed Vegetables and Brown Rice

Snack: Edamame Hummus with Whole Grain Pita Chips

DAY 4:

Breakfast: Mango Peach Smoothie

Lunch: Turkey and Avocado Wrap with Side Salad

Dinner: Baked Cod with Steamed Broccoli and Quinoa

Snack: Cucumber and Cream Cheese Roll-Ups

DAY 5:

Breakfast: Peanut Butter Banana Smoothie

Lunch: Lentil Soup with Whole Grain Bread

Dinner: Grilled Vegetable Skewers with Quinoa Pilaf

Snack: Roasted Chickpeas

DAY 6:

Breakfast: Mixed Berry and Spinach Smoothie

Lunch: Tuna Salad Lettuce Wraps

Dinner: Beef and Vegetable Stir-Fry with Brown Rice

Snack: Greek Yogurt Dip with Whole Grain Crackers

DAY 7:

Breakfast: Blueberry Banana Smoothie

Lunch: Chicken Caesar Salad with Whole Grain Croutons

Dinner: Eggplant Parmesan with Side Salad

Snack: Almond Flour Blueberry Muffins

DAY 8:
Breakfast: Tropical Paradise Smoothie
Lunch: Quinoa and Black Bean Salad
Dinner: Lemon Herb Grilled Chicken with Roasted Vegetables
Snack: Frozen Yogurt Bark with Mixed Nuts and Berries

DAY 9:
Breakfast: Creamy Avocado Smoothie
Lunch: Turkey and Vegetable Stir-Fry with Brown Rice
Dinner: Shrimp Scampi with Whole Wheat Pasta and Steamed Green Beans
Snack: Apple Slices with Almond Butter

DAY 10:
Breakfast: Raspberry Coconut Smoothie
Lunch: Greek Chicken Salad with Feta and Olives
Dinner: Vegetarian Chili with Cornbread
Snack: Caprese Skewers

DAY 11:

Breakfast: Greek Yogurt Parfait with Berries and Granola

Lunch: Hummus and Veggie Sticks

Dinner: Baked Salmon with Roasted Asparagus and Quinoa

Snack: Cottage Cheese with Pineapple

DAY 12:

Breakfast: Green Power Smoothie

Lunch: Caprese Salad with Grilled Chicken

Dinner: Stuffed Bell Peppers with Ground Turkey and Brown Rice

Snack: Edamame Hummus with Whole Grain Pita Chips

DAY 13:

Breakfast: Berry Blast Smoothie

Lunch: Greek Salad with Grilled Shrimp

Dinner: Chicken Stir-Fry with Mixed Vegetables and Brown Rice

Snack: Roasted Chickpeas

DAY 14:

Breakfast: Mango Peach Smoothie
Lunch: Turkey and Avocado Wrap with Side Salad
Dinner: Baked Cod with Steamed Broccoli and Quinoa
Snack: Cucumber and Cream Cheese Roll-Ups

Happy Cooking!

CONCLUSION

In conclusion, **"DASH Diet Meal Prep for Chronic Kidney Disease"** offers a comprehensive approach to managing CKD through mindful eating and meal preparation. By embracing the principles of the DASH Diet tailored specifically for kidney health, individuals with CKD can take control of their nutrition and enhance their overall well-being. Through understanding the importance of key nutrients, effective meal planning strategies, and a diverse array of delicious recipes, readers are empowered to make positive dietary choices that support kidney function and promote optimal health. Remember, this book is just the beginning of your journey towards a healthier lifestyle. With dedication, perseverance, and the guidance of healthcare professionals, you can navigate the challenges of CKD and thrive with nourishing, kidney-friendly meals. Let this book be your companion on the path to better health and vitality.

www.ingramcontent.com/pod-product-compliance
Lightning Source LLC
Chambersburg PA
CBHW050324230526
45471CB00005B/2342